THE BILLIONAIRE'S BOOK OF HEADACHES

THE BILLIONAIRE'S BOOK OF HEADACHES

Raeburn Forbes

Dedication

To Julie Anne and our children.

Contents

Acknowledgments

To all my clinical mentors from the start of my medical training in Dundee and to my colleagues today, including Dr. Rob Swingler, Sister Barbara Scott, Dr. Alastair Shaw, and Professor Ray Newton; Drs. Patterson, Gibson, Morrow, Watt, Esmonde, Hawkins, and Droogan in Belfast; my current colleagues, Drs. McKnight, Campbell, Rusk, and Wilson, and Dr. Gavin Briggs, neuroradiologist; and Dr. Manjit Matharu, London, for encouraging me in my specialist interest in headache. To the following physiotherapists for helping my understanding of the role of the neck in headache: Denise Hall, Julie Sugrue, and Rebecca Nelson. I am thankful for the administrative assistance of Hazel Neale of Craigavon Hospital Medical Library and Elaine Johnston, my secretary.

My name is Dr. Raeburn Forbes, and I'm a consultant neurologist who sees a lot of people with severe headaches. I entered the University of Dundee Medical School in 1987 and graduated MBChB and MD (Hons). I completed my training in adult neurology at the Royal Victoria Hospital in Belfast in July 2003, and in 2004 was appointed consultant neurologist in the Southern Health and Social Care Trust in Northern Ireland and started a private neurology practice.

I started writing SevereHeadacheExpert.com in August 2008, and since then, I have had more than five million website visitors. I wrote *The Billionaire's Book of Headaches* to help people make better choices about managing headaches. What you read is based on two decades of experience and is backed up by medical research (see the bibliography).

Many people become trapped by headaches and are on a search to discover the cause. If they knew the cause, then they would be able to fix the headache. However, the reasons for having headaches are complex. Headaches will return—research proves this.

An approach based on cause and effect will fail and frustrate. *The Billionaire's Book of Headaches* is for people who do not have a dangerous cause for their headaches. It takes a different approach to cause-and-effect thinking. What you read here is exactly what I would tell someone who had no limit on what they could spend.

I will show you why looking for migraine triggers is negative and damaging for your health. You will discover a free way of thinking that puts you in control. Severe headaches may have driven you into a lifestyle where you became trapped in patterns of negative thinking, such as "I can't stop thinking about my headaches."

Your life is controlled by headaches. You are no longer in charge. A key step to regaining control is understanding why you are in pain and accepting that this problem is part of who you are. You need to discover that you have control over how you respond to pain. My aim is to put you—the person with headache—back in control.

For some people, a series of fairly simple steps can greatly reduce the risk of headaches. For others, pain is present every day, no matter what. You'll be lucky to get fifteen minutes at a time with your doctor, and it's impossible to learn all you need to know in such a short time. Yet there is so much you can do!

I wrote *The Billionaire's Book of Headaches* to let you discover more at your own pace. Research proves that this information will reduce the number of headaches you get and the amount of medication used.

I hope that I can help you get back in control.

Raeburn Forbes, MD (Hons)
Consultant Neurologist
Author of *The Billionaire's Book of Headaches*
@raeburn
www.severe-headache-expert.com

Introduction

These days the rich seem to have everything and the rest of us make do. Imagine being a billionaire. Wouldn't life be great?

What if you also had headaches? What should you do if money was no object?

Welcome to *The Billionaire's Book of Headaches*. I want to save you time, money, and distress. This is what I'd tell billionaires who ask my advice on headaches - so you are not missing out.

Headaches cost the United States about $17 billion every year. Days off work and costs of treatment are huge. That's the money, but what about the cost to you? Pain and suffering. Lost time with friends and family. Unable to play or socialize. You can't put a price on that.

Traditional headache plans rely on looking for causes or triggers. You treat the cause. You hope for the effect—no headaches. You spend years looking for the cause. Yet your life is controlled by headaches.

Traditional headache plans are based on cause-and-effect thinking. Cause-and-effect thinking means you try to find out *why* you have headaches. Cause-and-effect thinking means you are forever looking for the reason for headaches. Cause-and-effect thinking means you need a diagnosis before you can treat. Cause-and-effect thinking means *you* are not in control—your headaches control you.

Searching for causes seems like a good idea. Everybody is doing it, and it seems to make sense. Maybe a food additive is causing your headaches? You check food labels or you ask the cook, "What's in the food?" You try hard to avoid the food additive. You hope for the effect—no headaches. With any luck you stop getting headaches. However, the effort of checking food labels has no end. You do this every day in case you get a headache. Then your next headache appears. What do you do now? You go looking for more causes. Looking for causes continues for years. You end up trapped by lists of things you *must* avoid. You're still thinking cause and effect.

No matter how hard you try, headaches *will* continue to happen. Swiss researchers followed several hundred headache sufferers for thirty years and found that an average headache sufferer has twenty-two days with headache every year. That's over fourteen hundred headaches in a lifetime. Were these people looking for causes? You bet they were—it's been the standard advice for decades.

If you can't stop headaches, you must change your thinking. Stop thinking cause and effect.

The Billionaire's Book of Headaches is a new way of dealing with headaches which will change your thinking and let you know the best way to control headaches. Your first step is to know that you are safe and do not have a dangerous headache. Seeing a doctor is the best way to rule out a dangerous headache. Dangerous headaches are completely new headaches, of recent onset, in someone who has never had headaches before. In dangerous headaches your eye examination or neurological examination may be abnormal. If you get a new onset headache, you must seek medical advice.

Once your doctor confirms that you are safe you're in a great position. See how you do not need an exact diagnosis? All you need is to know that you are safe. Knowing you are safe gives you freedom to try whatever you think helps your headaches. Knowing you are safe puts you in control.

Your second step is accepting your headaches. The Swiss researchers proved that people with headaches have an average of twenty-two days a year with headache. Acceptance sets you free from the endless search for causes or cures. It's not *if* a headache happens but *when*. Accepting headaches is not admitting defeat, it means changing your way of thinking. Your new aim is not to "cure" headaches. What you need is to live as well as you can—in spite of headaches.

Your third step is to ask, "How can I reduce my risk of headaches?" Take whatever steps you can to reduce the number and intensity of headaches. Focus on actions to make headaches less. *The Billionaire's Book of Headaches* shows you how to reduce your headache risk and common mistakes to avoid. Understand the best way to treat a headache attack, and how to use headache prevention medicines properly. Discover drug-free treatments and proven lifestyle changes that reduce your risk of headache. I want to challenge your thinking and show you how the 'law of migraine triggers' can trap you.

The Billionaire's Book of Headaches is based on years of experience and published research studies. Your doctor cannot teach you everything you need to know. You'll be lucky to get a fifteen-minute appointment. *The Billionaire's Book of Headaches* lets you find out more at your own pace. You have lots of options. This is all about you and how you can feel in control. Start reaping the rewards of headache research.

Fact: people who use information from research have fewer headaches.

Fact: people who use information from research use less medication.

Wishing you every success on your billionaire's journey.

Raeburn Forbes

Raeburn Forbes, MD (Hons)
Consultant Neurologist

How to Feel Safe

Headaches are dangerous, or they are not. When you've been told you're safe, it is really important you learn how to feel safe.

It's natural to feel afraid when you get a bad headache. Feeling afraid makes you pay more attention to pain. The more attention you pay to pain, the worse it gets. When pain keeps building, you wonder when it will end. When you feel safe and stop feeling afraid, pain is less likely to take over your life. Seeing your doctor, feeling safe, and understanding the pain system help you feel less afraid of headaches. When you understand the pain system, you will know the difference between good pain and bad pain.

The main reason to see your doctor is to rule out a dangerous headache. The actual diagnosis may not matter. You may need to make several visits to know you are OK. If your symptoms have changed, you may need to revisit the doctor after many years. The bottom line is that you need to feel safe. When you are safe, you pay less attention to pain and you feel less afraid.

Your body and brain have a network of nerves that stimulate fear, release adrenaline, and help you get out of trouble. This network is called the pain system. Fear makes you alert and wakens you to take action. Adrenaline makes your heart race so that you can fight or run away. If you are facing a physical danger, these emotional and bodily changes are helpful. The pain system helps you escape and seek help from others. These forces in your body and brain are powerful and difficult to resist. Once you escape danger, the pain system switches off and you feel relief.

Imagine your hand being too close to a fire. It starts to hurt. This pain makes you pull your hand away. This pain gets you out of trouble and stops you from getting burned. If you did get burned, then you would tell someone, "My hand hurts." The pain system is at its best when getting you away from a physical danger outside your body. This is good pain. Good pain has a purpose: it helps you survive, get out of trouble, and seek help.

When you suffer headaches, the pain system is activated again and again. You get the fear, adrenaline surge, anxiety, and stress as if you were facing a physical danger. You keep telling people about your headaches, and everyone gets more and more worried. But you cannot escape, as the symptoms are inside, not outside. When you cannot escape, your thinking changes, and you start to fear the next headache instead of feeling relief. You are trapped by headaches and cannot imagine a future where headaches are not in control. You think harmful thoughts: Will I have a stroke? Will my head burst? Do I have a brain tumor?

Although your headache is not dangerous, you feel all the negative emotions and memories that go along with pain. These fears and thoughts mean you have bad pain. Bad pain is pain without a purpose. Bad pain gives you trouble and does not help you escape. It's better to think of this bad pain as a false alarm.

Imagine a fire drill. The fire alarm goes off, and you get that adrenaline rush. When you realize there is no fire, you relax and go through the routine of the fire drill. Headaches are like a fire drill. When a headache begins, your instinct is to feel frightened and anxious. At that point you have a choice. You can let thoughts of danger take over, or you can start to think of this pain as a false alarm.

Practice feeling safe. Prepare yourself physically and mentally for headaches. Be ready with treatments to take and know how to distract yourself from the pain. Distractions help your body avoid the unpleasant feelings that accompany pain. Distractions take attention away from pain and make it easier to cope.

If you don't feel safe, headaches and fear take over. If you feel you're in danger, you struggle to cope. You won't be able to think of anything else. Headaches become your main focus and ruin your life.

Understand how the pain system works so that you can feel less afraid of pain. Make sure your doctor has examined you so that you can feel safe. Fight the negative thoughts and emotions that headaches bring.

When you feel safe, it is much easier to accept your headaches. When you know you are safe, you have the freedom to try whatever you think is reasonable to make your life better. You no longer have the worry that something bad is about to happen, and you are free to take steps to reduce your risk of headache.

The next chapter explains common headache types and non-headache symptoms. Understanding your symptoms and knowing what to expect helps you feel safe and in control.

The Billionaire's Book of Headaches is your path to getting in control. When you feel safe, accept your headaches, and start reducing risk, headaches can no longer get the better of you. Whatever you do, you must always make sure you are safe and feel safe.

2

What Type of Headache Is Mine?

(understanding your symptoms helps you feel safe)

In *The Billionaire's Book of Headaches*, you need to follow this way of thinking:

- Know that you are *safe*.
- *Accept* your headaches.
- *Reduce your risk* of headaches.

Becoming familiar with symptoms makes them less worrisome and helps you feel safe. You must know more about the common head-ache types and which non-headache symptoms occur.

Most headache episodes last between six and twenty-four hours. Some headaches last for weeks and then go away again. If you get a headache every day (or only occasional pain-free days), your brain cannot switch off pain. This faulty off switch means that pain continues or returns very often. In almost everyone this is not a sign of disease, it is just the way your brain is made.

Your headache type depends on how you describe the headache and on having a normal eye and neurological examination. Your family doctor or general practitioner can confirm tension-type headache, migraine, ice pick headache, and chronic migraine. A neurologist, headache specialist, or brain scans are not normally required for these common headache types.

Notice that it's not *headache diagnosis* but *headache type*.

Why?

If you do not have a dangerous headache, the steps you take are exactly the same, with very few exceptions. [1] A good rule is to manage bad headaches, which are not dangerous, as migraine. Don't get stuck on diagnosis. It is much better to accept that you are someone with headaches who is safe and needs to reduce the risk of headache.

Next, let's look at each of the most common headache types so that you can start to feel safe.

TENSION-TYPE HEADACHE

Tension-type headache causes you feel a tight band or pressure in or around your head. Some say it's like a weight on top of the head or squeezing around the head. Tension-type headache occurs in any location—top, side, back, front, or all around the head.

---

1 Some of the rare headache disorders such as cluster headache and trigeminal neuralgia have very specific treatments that are different from migraine. Dangerous headaches have their own treatments specific to each condition.

Tension-type headache can occur on one side or both and may switch sides. Most people say tension-type headache is a nuisance and not severe. Most people manage tension-type headache without seeing a doctor: "It's just a headache." Tension-type headache does not usually stop you from doing what you want to do. An episode of tension-type headache can last from a few hours to days or weeks.

About one in three people have at least one episode of tension-type headache a year, so it's the most common headache type known. People who experience tension-type headache more than fifteen days per month have chronic tension-type headache.[2]

MIGRAINE HEADACHE

Migraine is more severe than tension-type headache. Your head may throb slowly at about forty beats per minute. Not every one with migraine feels throbbing pain. Many people cannot put migraine headache into words: "It's just very sore."

For others, migraine headache is sharp or feels like a pressure that is much more intense than tension-type headache. Migraine headache affects one side of the head more than the other but can affect both sides at the same time. Some people have side-locked migraine—it's only on one side of the head and never the other. Some people get migraine over the front of the head or only around the eye, but any location is possible.

---

2 People who are overweight (body mass index greater than thirty) with chronic tension-type headache must ensure they do not have idiopathic intracranial hypertension, which is usually ruled out by an eye examination, visual field test, and lumbar puncture test.

The main difference between migraine and tension-type headache is the presence of one or more of these six symptoms:

1. You feel nauseous or off food.
2. You prefer the dark, as the headache is made worse by light.
3. You avoid noise and prefer quietness.
4. Strong smells make you feel awful.
5. Movement makes the pain worse, so you want to lie still.
6. Your head feels too sore to touch.

These are the six symptoms of sensory sensitivity. People with migraine have two or more of these symptoms, along with headache. People with migraine prefer to lie down in dark and quiet spaces and do not want to continue normal activities. This is different from tension-type headache, where you typically continue normal activity in spite of the pain, and sensory sensitivity symptoms are usually absent or very mild.

During a migraine you can feel dizzy or find it difficult to concentrate, as if the brain has completely slowed down or is in a fog. Although annoying and even frightening, this is normal for migraine.

Many people with migraine have face pain or feel like pain is in their sinuses. About 25 percent of people can get a runny nose or watery eyes during a migraine headache. This can lead to a belief that the problem is a sinus headache. People with sinus headache, which does not respond to sinus treatment, usually have migraine. If you think the sinus is the cause of your headache, then you may put yourself through unnecessary sinus treatments.

Your eye and neurological examinations are normal in migraine.

One in six women and one in twelve men get migraine headache at some point in their lives. Migraine is the most common type of headache that makes people want to visit a doctor. Non-headache symptoms accompany migraine headache and are called migraine aura and the migraine prodrome.

MIGRAINE AURA

Twenty percent of people with migraine headache get migraine aura. Migraine aura causes you to experience brain symptoms, such as visual disturbance, tingling, weakness, speech disturbance, or vertigo, which can happen at any time. Migraine aura starts just before (or at the same time as) a migraine headache. Migraine aura spreads over several minutes, lasts for about an hour, and then goes away completely. The symptoms are often mistaken for a stroke, which is frightening if you do not understand migraine aura.

Migraine aura may happen without any headache and usually starts before pain appears. Migraine aura is due to a random reduction in brain activity called cortical spreading depression, which slowly shuts down the brain's natural electrical activity, thus causing the symptoms to appear. Usually within an hour or two, the brain wakes up again and the symptoms settle.

Migraine aura symptoms in people with migraine who have a normal examination by their doctors and opticians do not need their symptoms investigated. Migraine aura must be investigated in people who have *never* had any headache (this is called isolated migraine aura).

When you know which headache and non-headache symptoms are typical for migraine, it's easier to feel safe, and feeling safe helps you cope with pain.

THE MIGRAINE PRODROME

The migraine prodrome occur hours before migraine headache and includes hunger, thirst, depression, a sense of doom, elation, feeling full of energy, cravings for specific foods, fatigue, lethargy, or irritability. Many people know a migraine headache is on its way because of the migraine prodrome. Some people cannot put the migraine prodrome into words: "I just know I'm going to get a migraine."

Food cravings are a symptom of migraine prodrome. You can be fooled into thinking that your migraine is caused by specific foods. More likely it's the migraine prodrome making you want the food. The food is not causing the migraine—it's the other way round. The migraine is making you want the food.

Now you know that there is a wide range of symptoms that people with migraine can experience—sensory sensitivity symptoms, migraine aura, and migraine prodrome—and that it's not just about pain.

ICE PICK HEADACHE

Imagine you have been stabbed in the head with a spike—that's what an ice pick headache feels like. An ice pick headache disappears quickly, lasting no more than a few seconds. A severe ice pick headache may make you grab your head or feel weak at the knees.

Ice pick headache can settle into a mild pain that feels like tension-type headache for a few minutes or hours. An ice pick headache may intensify into a typical migraine headache. This can happen if you get several ice pick headaches one after the other. Some people get a sudden sharp pain that persists at a severe level for up to a minute, which can feel terrifying.

Ice pick headache is usually in or around the eye but can happen in any part of the head or neck. It can feel like a line running through your head from back to front or top to bottom. Ice pick headaches are more common in people with tension-type headache and migraine, but some people get only ice pick headaches.

Ice pick headache is confirmed by a typical medical history and normal neurological and eye examinations. Brain scans are not needed if your neurological and eye examinations are normal.

COMBINATIONS OF HEADACHE TYPES

It is normal to get different types of headache. Some people get only tension-type headache and never get migraine. Some people get only migraine and never get tension-type headache. Some people have migraine headache one year and then tension-type headache the next year. Many people get both. Research shows that any combination of tension-type headache, migraine headache, or ice pick headache is possible. It is best to think of yourself as someone with recurring headaches who is safe rather than getting stuck on the actual name of the headache. If a headache feels bad enough to treat, then you treat it like a migraine.

The group of people with the largest number of headaches and the widest range of non-headache symptoms usually has chronic migraine.

CHRONIC MIGRAINE

Each year about one in fifty migraine sufferers changes from episodes of migraine headache into chronic migraine. With chronic migraine, headaches become more frequent, until the head is never clear of pain or you have only an occasional pain-free day. There is a continuous background headache, which feels like tension-type headache or a mild migraine.

On top of this background headache, you experience a lot of severe migraine headaches, maybe every day or at least once a week. Among these different headaches, you experience several sensory sensitivity symptoms, migraine aura, or migraine prodrome symptoms. You can also get headaches that feel like tension-type or ice pick headaches.

With chronic migraine, there is no symptom pattern. It is one thing after another.

With chronic migraine, your head is a ball of chaos.

A key symptom of chronic migraine is heightened sensitivity to touch, light, noise, or smell. Brushing or washing your hair or scalp can feel unbearable. You want to avoid light every day or wear dark glasses to feel more comfortable. It can feel like any noise is agony, and a slight smell makes you feel sick.

If you do not understand the symptoms of chronic migraine, you get distressed. Distress makes pain worse and drives you to take extreme measures. Symptoms are so frequent that you are desperate to find patterns, or triggers. This is cause-and-effect thinking, and it's a bad idea. There is no pattern to find, except that the symptoms keep on coming.

In *The Billionaire's Book of Headaches*, I'm trying to put you back in control by letting you know what can happen if you suffer frequent headaches. When you know the range of symptoms you can experience, you start to feel safe.

Instead of thinking, "My headache diagnosis is...," think instead, "I get different headache types, which are not dangerous" or "I get headaches, but I am safe."

When you feel safe, it is easier to accept your headaches. Then you can take whatever steps you wish to reduce your headache risk. This approach saves you time and a lot of distress.

Next, we look at the number one way you can reduce the risk of headaches. Are you overusing painkillers?

3

Why Taking Too Many Painkillers Makes Things Worse

(and what to do about it)

Taking painkillers over ten days per month increases the risk of bad headaches. If you do this, it's not your fault. It's human nature to do whatever it takes to get rid of pain, but you could be doing more harm than good.

When you have bad headaches and take too many painkillers, the official diagnosis is medication overuse headache. However, this diagnosis itself is misleading.

A diagnosis of medication overuse headache suggests that the painkillers caused the headache. If overusing painkillers caused headaches, then stopping the painkillers would stop the headaches. This is not true. Fifty percent of people who stop their painkillers *continue* to get severe headaches. The good news is that 50 percent of people who stop painkillers go from bad headaches every day to being pain-free most of the time.

A diagnosis of medication overuse headache is based on cause-and-effect thinking. It is better to realize that overusing painkillers *increases the risk of headaches*. The opposite is true. Reducing painkillers *reduces the risk of headaches*. Please understand that stopping painkillers does not cure your headaches. That is cause-and-effect thinking, and it leads to disappointment.

However, a 50 percent chance of reducing your risk of headaches is one that you must take. Everyone who has problem headaches must try to stop all painkillers.

Stopping painkillers is hard to do, so you must know what to expect. Before you try to stop, you need to get your thinking straight. You must understand what I mean by *reducing risk* as opposed to *dealing with the cause*.

Let's compare risk with cause. Imagine driving your car very fast. Another car pulls out in front of you. You can't avoid the other car, so you crash. The other driver was at fault, as he or she pulled out in front you, and you could not react in time. Yet by driving too fast, you *increased the risk* of a crash. If you were driving slower, you still might have crashed, but you would have had more time to react. Driving fast *increased the risk* of crashing. Driving more slowly would have *reduced the risk* of crashing.

Taking too many painkillers does not cause headaches, and stopping painkillers will not cure headaches. If you try to stop painkillers while engaging in cause-and-effect thinking, then you will end up frustrated. Taking too many painkillers increases the risk of head-aches. If you stop overusing painkillers, you reduce the risk of head-aches. In one study, the risk of bad headaches was twenty-five times higher in people who overused painkillers. You need to know that you are trying to reduce your risk of headaches, not cure them.

When you stop painkillers, your headaches feel worse for a few weeks. This worsening (of already bad headaches) is called rebound headache. When your headache gets worse, you think your doc-tor got it wrong. You felt better *on* the painkillers. Within days you restart the painkillers. You make the mistake of thinking that pain-killers were helping you after all. In the short term, taking painkillers feels better than taking none. But this is how you get caught in the trap of painkiller overuse. In the long term, this makes it more likely you will have bad headaches.

The first two weeks of stopping painkillers can be awful, especially the first few days, when you feel like there is nothing you can do (see the account of stopping painkillers in appendix 2). Other symptoms occur during rebound headaches, such as restlessness, nausea, vom-iting, and tremor. You get very strong feelings that you *must* have painkillers. It feels bad because your brain and body have been used to painkillers for a long time. The brain responds to stopping drugs by making you feel sore and uncomfortable—your brain still wants the drugs.

You need to allow your brain time to rest and to reset itself. This means avoiding the original painkillers for at least four weeks, and better still, eight weeks—the longer, the better. People feel guilty about overusing painkillers and try to hide it from family or friends. It's so easy to get caught in the cycle of headaches and painkillers. You should not blame yourself for the painkiller problem. It's human nature to seek out a solution to pain.

If you are one of the 50 percent of people who improve, research shows that you may reduce your number of headaches by 50 percent. So if you were getting twenty headaches a month, you may reduce that to ten a month. This is a massive difference. Notice how this is not 100 percent—there will still be some headaches—but you have reduced your risk.

When you stop overusing painkillers, it feels frightening to think of going days or weeks without them. Your doctor can prescribe a bridging treatment, such as steroids or anti-inflammatory drugs. These might reduce the risk of rebound headaches but must only be taken under medical supervision. These bridging treatments are started on the same day that you stop your painkillers and are taken every day for between five and fourteen days. During this time expect to feel worse before you get better, and be determined not to restart your old painkillers once more. In appendix 2, the diary shows how a bridging treatment is used when you try to stop painkillers.

Guidelines on managing headaches recommend you stop painkillers all at once rather than withdraw the dose slowly. It is possible to do a bit of both. If you have used high doses of strong painkillers for a long time, you may feel better reducing slowly to a lower dose. Once on a lower dose, you stop everything. If you are going to stop painkillers, please discuss this with your doctor first. Be safe and feel safe.

Stopping painkillers, if you overuse them, is the best way to reduce your risk of headache. Specialist headache centers always make sure painkillers are stopped first, which sometimes requires admission for a week or more. Specialist headache centers will not consider advanced treatments for headaches until they know you have tried stopping painkillers—it's that important.

If you understand medication withdrawal and rebound headaches, then you can feel in control. Feeling in control means feeling safe. When you feel safe, it's easier to push through and to stop overusing painkillers.

By now you should have some idea of what sort of symptoms to expect when you get headaches and why stopping painkillers is the number one step you must take if you struggle with headaches.

Remember that the process of *The Billionaire's Book of Headaches* is to

- feel safe;
- accept your headaches; and
- reduce your risk of headaches.

It's about avoiding common errors, being smart with your medication, and adding in positive lifestyle changes. It's no longer about finding causes and cures. It's all about reducing your risk, and one of the biggest ways to reduce risk is to stop overusing painkillers. In the next chapter, find out how to treat a headache with medicines without falling into the trap of medication overuse.

4

How to Treat a Headache with Medicines

(without overusing them)

The best way to go about treating a headache episode is to assume that you are treating a migraine. Remember that migraine and the other common headache types are not a sign of serious disease—you are safe, no matter how much pain you feel.

Research shows us smart ways to treat migraine headache:

- There is a gap at the start of a headache when medicines work best.
- Combinations work better than single medicines.
- Use distractions alongside medicines.
- Be prepared for a headache return.

It's important to plan for another headache. Our Swiss researchers proved that it's an average of twenty-two days per year with headaches for people like you. Headaches *will* happen.

If you engage in cause-and-effect thinking, you focus on avoiding or removing *causes* to get to the point of never having a headache. You believe that one day headaches will stop. This prevents you from preparing for what to do when a headache happens.

Waiting rooms, doctors' offices, and emergency rooms are unpleasant places when you have a bad headache, with their bright lights, noises, and odors. You're waiting for someone else, and you are not in control. You must feel in control. If you have a headache plan, you should be able to manage headaches at home. A billionaire would have a comfortable, quiet, dark, and relaxing area to see him or her through a bad headache—the billionaire's bunker!

THE GAP AT THE START OF A HEADACHE

When you get a migraine headache, pain usually builds up from nothing (0 out of 10) to maximum pain (10 out of 10) in about one to two hours. Some are quicker, and some are slower. Some get to 10 out of 10, and some do not. If you get a lot of headaches, then your past experience will tell you what to expect.

Somewhere in between 0 and 10 you need to take action. Do you wait until the pain is 9 out of 10? Do you get in at 1 out at 10? Which is better? When treating a headache with migraine medicines, research tells us that they work best *before your head is too sore to touch*.

When normal touch becomes painful, this is called allodynia. Pain-sensitive nerves switching into an overactive state cause allodynia.

With allodynia, your head feels tender and sore to move. Allodynia means you avoid brushing or washing your hair because it's too sore. People with headaches usually know exactly when allodynia happens.

Allodynia may happen when pain is mild, so there is a shorter gap to use medicines. Allodynia may not happen until pain is more severe, so there is a longer gap to use medicines. Some people never get allodynia. By the time allodynia happens, treatment works about 10 to 20 percent of the time. Before allodynia, the chance of reducing pain within two to four hours is closer to 70 percent.

This is a huge difference. This is a great way of using research to *reduce your headache risk.*

To treat a headache, try to use migraine medicines before your head is too sore to touch. Remember that there is a gap at the start of a headache when medicines work best.

Sometimes, no matter what you do, a headache continues. It is possible to treat before allodynia and not see a response. Nothing is 100 percent guaranteed. If nothing is working, make yourself as comfortable as possible, go to bed, and rest or sleep until the headache eases. There will be times when all you can do is weather the storm.

If you do not already know, try to find out at what level of headache you reach allodynia. Learn to treat a headache before allodynia sets in.

USE COMBINATIONS OF MEDICINES

When headaches are bad enough to need medicines, combinations of medicines work better than each on its own. Think of headache medicines in groups: group A (anti-inflammatory painkillers), group B (triptans), and group C (anti-sickness). Within each group there is very little to choose from between each medicine. If a particular medicine from one group works, then stick to it. If one doesn't work, then try another from that group. In most countries these are prescription-only medicines that should only be used following advice from your doctor or pharmacist.

Group A: Painkillers

Soluble aspirin (Ecotrin, Bufferin), ibuprofen (Advil, Motrin), naproxen (Aleve, Naprosyn), tolfenamic acid (NSAIDs), acetaminophen (Tylenol, Panadol)

Group B: Triptans

Sumatriptan (Imitrex, Zecuity), zolmitriptan (Zomig, Zomig-ZMT), rizatriptan (Maxalt, Maxalt-MLT), almotriptan (Axert), frovatriptan (Frova), naratriptan (Amerge), eletriptan (Relpax)

Group C: Anti-sickness

Metoclopramide (Reglan, Metozolv ODT), prochlorperazine (Compro, Prochlorperazine Edisylate Novaplus), cyclizine (antihistamine), domperidone (Motilium)

You choose one medicine from group A and one medicine from group B, and if you get nausea, you choose a medicine from group C.[3]

As soon as you feel the pain building, and *before your head is too sore to touch*, you take A + B + C together. If you don't get much nausea, you could hold off using C. While you wait for these medicines to work, distract yourself from the pain. If you can, lie down and sleep awhile. Sleep can help refresh your brain if you suffer from headaches.

With bodily pain, a doctor recommends starting painkillers low and building them up only if pain increases. For some reason, headaches, especially migraines, are different from bodily pain. You have to hit headaches hard and early. Use combinations, and remember the gap at the start when your chance of success is greatest.

USE DISTRACTIONS

Distractions are important. The more attention you give pain, the worse it feels. You can bring on a headache by thinking about the *possibility* of pain. Prepare distractions to put into action when a headache appears.

Common distractions include walking or brief vigorous exercise (e.g., a sprint on an exercise bike); listening to or playing music; reading

---

3 These are not the only medicines in each group. Others exist, and the choice depends on local prescribing practice and medicine availability.

poetry; writing; relaxation techniques, including meditation, yoga, mindfulness, and prayer; applying hot or cold towels to the head and neck; and controlled breathing techniques called biofeedback.

After about twenty-four hours, you should, on average, be getting to the end of a headache attack. Surveys show that an average migraine headache lasts twenty-four hours. If you routinely get headaches lasting several days, you need to be certain you do not have an issue with medication overuse. Persistent headaches are also a good reason to check your eyes, neck, jaw, or sleep habits, all of which are covered in other chapters.

If a headache persists, be careful about continuing more medication, or you increase the risk of medication overuse. You can repeat your medicines (A + B + C) once within twenty-four hours, and most people want to repeat between four and eight hours. If your headache is unusually sore or persistent, remember to consult your doctor if nothing is working as you expect.

Try to limit painkillers to an average of ten days per month, or you will increase the risk of headaches worsening. Notice the word *average*. If you have one month with five days of painkiller use and the next month with fifteen days of painkiller use, that is an average of ten days each month. There is a lot of variation in headache frequency, so having some months with more and some months with less is OK. Just be aware that using painkillers on a majority of days can make headaches worse, and you should try to limit the amount you use.

Do not feel ashamed or that it is your fault that you need painkillers. Using a lot of painkillers is not a sign of addiction. It is just a sign that you are not coping well and need to consider as many different strategies as possible to help you live well in spite of headaches.

Distractions help you use fewer painkillers and reduce the risk of overuse. Feeling safe and understanding your headache symptoms also help reduce use of medicines. This is why you need *The Billionaire's Book of Headaches*. It's not just about having a list of drugs. You must understand more about what pain means. You should change your thinking so that you feel safe. When your thinking is correct, medicines have the best chance of working.

THE HEADACHE RETURN

For a few hours, you may start to feel pain settling down, but after four hours, the pain can build up again. This happens in about 50 percent of cases and is called a headache return. If you don't know about headache return, you can feel like your treatment has failed. You can worry that things are getting out of control or something very bad is happening. If you get a headache return after four hours, just repeat your A + B + C. Knowing about headache return helps you feel less frightened. A second use of A + B + C reduces the risk of a headache running on for several days.

Talk to your doctor about having an emergency stock of your A + B + C drugs available at home. Write out an action plan for treating headaches. Remember which distractions you have chosen. Be prepared for a headache return, and if all else fails, you just have to weather the storm (in your billionaire's bunker).

Appendix 3 provides an example of using distractions and treating a headache episode with A + B + C.

Research shows that people with headaches use fewer medicines and report fewer headaches when they understand more about their headache problem: knowledge is power when you are dealing with headaches.

Remember *The Billionaire's Book of Headaches* approach:

- Feel safe.
- Accept your headaches.
- Reduce risk.

If you need to treat a headache more than twice a week, you may need headache prevention medicines. The next chapter shows you the common errors to avoid and how to use headache prevention medicines to reduce the risk of headache.

5

How to Use Headache Prevention Medicines

(use the best dose, and don't give up)

If you have headaches more than twice a week, you should consider using a headache prevention medicine. These medicines reduce your headache risk as long as one of your headache types is migraine. There are many different headache prevention medicines. Regardless of the one you use, the advice on how to start, monitor, and end treatment is the same.

Here's how to make the most of headache prevention medicines:

- Know what to expect.
- Understand why you shouldn't stop too soon.
- Keep a headache diary.
- Know the best dose to use.
- Understand what to do if medicines don't work.

The most commonly prescribed medicines are pizotifen (Sandomigran), propranolol (Inderal, InnoPran XL), amitriptyline (Elavil, Vanatrip), and topiramate (Topamax, Trokendi XR). Other preventive medicines can be bought without prescription, such as feverfew, magnesium, and vitamin B2.

KNOW WHAT TO EXPECT

The best dose of a successful headache prevention medicine reduces the number of headache episodes by about 30 percent, and some people see a reduction of at least 50 percent. Any headache that does appear may feel less severe or not be as long. Most people do not become headache-free, but you can get a good spell lasting many months. At some point headaches will return, but do not look for a cure. Don't get distracted by cause-and-effect thinking. You are trying to reduce your risk of headaches, not cure them.

When using headache prevention medicines, some people start to feel more tension-type headaches instead of migraine. It can feel a bit strange if the type of headache changes from migraine to tension-type headache, but this is normal. Remember that most people get combinations of headache types, and the combinations you get may change when you take headache prevention medicines. You should see it as a success if you have less of the severe headaches but more of the milder headaches. When you use headache prevention medicines, you aim to reduce headache risk, but your pattern of headache types may alter.

WHY YOU SHOULD NOT STOP TOO SOON

Within days or weeks of starting headache prevention medicines, another headache may happen. Do not give up if this occurs. Do not fall into cause-and-effect thinking. Another headache is not a failure. Another headache is not a sign that a medicine is not working. Here's why you must not give up.

Research shows that headache prevention medicines work by making the brain less reactive to physical energy like light, noise, or movement. A best dose of a headache prevention medicine takes twelve weeks before the brain fully adjusts and becomes less reactive. Imagine having ten days of headache in a month before starting a headache prevention medicine. If you aim to reduce your risk of headache by 50 percent, it might take three months of using a best dose of medicine before your headaches reduce to five per month. It is possible that in month one or two that you could still have had just as many headaches as when you started. It takes about twelve weeks of using a best dose of medicine before you notice a reduction in headaches. If you have no response after twelve weeks of using the best dose of a headache prevention medicine, then you need to try another.

When you use headache prevention medicines, you are trying to reduce your risk of headaches, not cure them. Have a realistic idea of what to expect, as it takes time. It is a very common mistake to give up too soon.

KEEP A HEADACHE DIARY

A headache diary is the simplest way to judge the effect of medicines on headaches. A headache diary is a simple record that lets you measure the number of headaches before and after a treatment. All you need to do is write down a number on a scale between 0 and 10 for your pain that day. Zero means no pain, and 10 means the worst pain you can imagine. What you are trying to do is work out if the overall amount of headache reduces.

Always record painkiller use in your diary. Remember that you are trying to limit painkillers to an average of ten days per month. Note the word *average*. If one month you have fifteen days of use and the next month is five days of use, then your average is ten days.

Keep a headache diary for four weeks before you start a new treatment. This gives you a starting point. For the last four weeks of a best dose, keep another headache diary. Compare the two headache diaries. Were there fewer headaches in the last four weeks than before you started? Did you reduce your risk of headache? Did you feel better and more able to live a normal life?

Expensive smartphone apps or devices that encourage you to record several triggers are not necessary. They push you back into cause-and-effect thinking. You are better off to accept your headaches and to focus on reducing risk. Use the diary in appendix 4 at the back of this book.

If you have decided to use headache prevention medicines, then you need to know that there is usually a best dose for each person.

KNOW THE BEST DOSE TO USE

Some people cope with big doses of drugs, but others get side effects with small doses. The best dose is somewhere between the starting dose and the maximum allowed. The best dose is the highest dose of medicine you can tolerate for a minimum of three months. If a drug gives you unpleasant side effects, then it is at too high a dose or it is not for you. You need to stick with a best dose for at least three months to get the full benefit, and remember that your aim is to reduce the risk of headaches, not cure them.

You find your best dose by slowly increasing the headache prevention medicine every week. Keep going until you reach as much as you can tolerate or the maximum dose allowed. It is OK if you cannot reach the maximum dose allowed. Your best dose may be *less* than the maximum allowed. It's better to run a lower dose you can tolerate for twelve weeks than to take nothing at all. An example of finding a best dose is presented in appendix 5.

Remember to keep a headache diary. This is the only way to know if you are reducing your risk of headache. If your diary has shown that you are reducing your risk of headache, then stick with your best dose for another six months.

When using headache prevention medicines, you are committing to almost a year of medicines every day. It may take a month to find your best dose and another three months to know if the best dose has worked. You should then continue for another six months if your headaches have reduced. That's a total of ten months just to test one medicine! Always review your use of headache prevention medicines with your doctor at the end of a year. If you stop headache prevention medicines after a year, you may get many months without needing to go back on them again, as the prevention effect persists after the medicines are stopped. Do not be disappointed if headaches increase again—at some point they probably will. You just start again with the same drug or try another one.

Headache prevention medicines are not linked with medication overuse headache. Medication overuse headache is only a problem with the painkillers you take at the time of a headache episode. Using painkillers every day increases the risk of headache, but using headache prevention medicines every day reduces the risk of headache.

WHAT TO DO IF MEDICINES DON'T WORK

If one medicine doesn't work, try another. You may need to try three different medicines before you find one that suits you. If three different headache prevention medicines have not reduced your headaches, then you likely have chronic migraine. If you just cannot tolerate any medicines, then your best option is to look at all the drug-free options discussed later in this book.

With chronic migraine, you could try more headache prevention medicines, but the chance of success is reduced if the three best-dose medicines have not worked. Some people who do not respond to headache prevention medicine have a physical illness that makes headaches worse, such as anemia, obstructive sleep apnea, or endocrine disease (e.g., thyroid, adrenal, or pituitary).

In addition to headache prevention medicines, it is important to consider the drug-free options. Could treating your neck, jaw, or eyes reduce your headache risk?

6

Check Your Neck, Jaw, and Eyes

(drug-free treatments to reduce headache risk)

If you have neck pain or stiffness, you increase your risk of headache fivefold. Jaw symptoms increase headache risk sevenfold. Adults with eye problems (shortsighted) are at double the risk of headache. If you engage in cause-and-effect thinking, you may be fooled into believing that treating the neck, using a mouth guard, or getting new glasses may cure your headache.

It's better to see neck, jaw, and eye treatments as ways to reduce your risk of headache. Better still, these treatments are drug-free.

THE NECK

Research involving thousands of people shows that headaches are five times more common in people with frequent neck pain or stiffness. The neck pain or stiffness does not have to be severe, it just has to be frequent. Forty to 70 percent of people with migraine get pain or stiffness in the neck during a headache episode. Many people with migraine rub or apply something cool to the neck to get relief. Headaches and neck aches are closely linked.

Your brain cannot tell the difference between neck pain and head pain, and one pain can make you feel the other. The reason for this is that the nerves in the upper neck and the nerves that sense pain from the head join together before they reach the surface of the brain.[4] Many people with neck problems report headache, and most people with headaches experience neck pain.

Researchers in Italy did an experiment with office workers. Some offices were taught to take a twice-daily break from work to exercise the neck, jaw, and shoulders. The other offices did not do the exercises. People in the offices who did the exercises reduced their headaches from an average of seven per month to five per month, a 30 percent reduction. The offices with no exercises had no change in headache risk. Paying attention to exercising the neck, jaw, and shoulders reduced the risk of headache.

Most people with neck pain and headache do not have a disease of the neck. What they have is stiffness from joints, muscles, and ligaments called cervical spine hypomobility.

One research study found cervical spine hypomobility in over 75 percent of people with headache. Most people with cervical spine hypomobility do not realize that they have this problem or that it increases the risk of headache. If your neck is not examined properly, cervical spine hypomobility remains undetected.

---

4 This group of nerves is called the trigeminocervical convergence.

Trigger points are very sensitive areas of skin and muscle, and if you have them in your neck, they may also increase headache risk. Like cervical spine hypomobility, they are found only when your neck is examined. A physiotherapist can help you identify trigger points and show you how to massage them gently to make them less sensitive. This can help reduce headache risk.

Previous neck injury (like whiplash) or head injury (like concussion) are common in people with cervical spine hypomobility. Neck problems also happen to students and desk workers with bad posture habits. The Paris physician Dr. Robert Maigne described cervical spine hypomobility in the 1950s. Dr. Maigne's observations are published only in French, and they are just now becoming mainstream in English-speaking countries. Osteopaths and physiotherapists have claimed success in treating headache, as their treatments increase neck mobility and reduce risk of headache.

Most people with headache and neck pain who see a doctor are told they have migraine or tension-type headache. Neck and shoulder exercises or hands-on treatment by a physiotherapist or osteopath can unblock neck stiffness. This leads to a reduction in headache risk. Even better is to learn how to look after your own neck so that you are not dependent on having someone treat it. You can learn how to release your own trigger points through gentle massage or to increase neck mobility with exercises to the upper parts of the cervical spine. This keeps you in control.

Treating the neck does not cure your headache—that is cause-and-effect thinking. Neck treatment, including exercises you can do yourself, *reduces your risk* of headache. As these treatments are drug-free, you must consider them—you have nothing to lose.

About 70 percent of people I send to physiotherapists notice that their risk of headache is reduced by up to 50 percent. Clinical trials of people with frequent headaches and abnormal neck examinations also show similar reductions in pain over several months. These people are not rid of headache, but they have reduced their risk of headache.

Everyone with frequent headaches should seek advice from a qualified physiotherapist (physical therapist) or reputable osteopath. You should ask for advice on how to exercise your neck. If you have cervical spine hypomobility, courses of controlled neck manipulation can help reduce headache risk. You should avoid high-velocity maneuvers that suddenly crack neck joints, as these may be harmful.

THE JAW

The jaw joint and jaw muscles are connected to the same nerve as the rest of your head, which is called the trigeminal nerve. Jaw joints and jaw muscles send pain signals to your brain and *increase your risk* of headache. People with jaw symptoms are seven times more likely to experience migraine or tension-type headaches than people without jaw symptoms.

Exercises to keep your jaw joint mobile reduce headache frequency. You can exercise the jaw by opening and closing the jaw against gentle pressure ten times twice a day. Some dentists offer appliances to prevent you from clenching your teeth during sleep. Prolonged jaw clenching increases the risk of headaches. Clenching your jaw during sleep also causes snoring, which can lead to daytime tiredness and increase the risk of headache. Dental appliances relax jaw muscles, which reduces tension in the muscles and stops snoring.

If your jaw muscles and joints are relaxed, you reduce your risk of headaches. In one study, a jaw appliance was found to reduce headaches by 46 percent after five months of use. Once again note that they did not cure the headaches.

The following questions may help you identify a potential problem with your jaw:

- Do you experience jaw pain or stiffness upon wakening?
- Do you experience jaw pain lasting for up to a week at a time?
- Do any of the following activities bring on jaw pain?
  - Chewing hard on tough food
  - Opening your mouth or moving your jaw to the side
  - Clenching your jaw or teeth or chewing gum
  - Talking, yawning, or kissing

If you answered yes to most of these questions, then part of your problem may be your jaw joint or jaw muscles, and you should visit your dentist.

Ask your dentist about jaw exercises or a jaw appliance as a drug-free way to reduce the risk of headache.

THE EYES

People with short sight increase their risk of headache by at least twice that of people who are not shortsighted. Refractive errors, which are the common type of short sight, are more frequent in people with migraine than in people without migraine.

There are three ways eye problems increase headache risk:

1. The muscles that focus your lens (ciliary muscles) send pain signals to your brain, which you feel as a headache.
2. Peering forward to get a better view causes a mild neck strain that sends pain signals to your head (so the eye is making you strain your neck).
3. Distortion of the visual image causes overactivity in the surface of your brain, leading to migraine headache.

Having your optician correct an eye abnormality can reduce headache risk. Opticians can also carefully examine the inside of your eye.

An optician may see signs of increased brain fluid pressure called papilloedema. Papilloedema is rare—a one in ten thousand chance—but if found requires an urgent brain scan, which may be lifesaving. Signs of other medical diseases can be picked up by an optician, such as diabetes, glaucoma, and high blood pressure. You have nothing to lose by seeing an optician. At the very least, you will see better. If your examination does not show signs of serious disease, then it is another way to know that you are safe.

The Billionaire's Book of Headaches is not just about medicines. Improving your neck, jaw, or eyes can reduce your risk of headache. Just like any other treatment, you should keep a headache diary to see if improving your neck, jaw, or eyes is having any effect. You have nothing to lose.

Remember:

- Feel safe.
- Accept your headaches.
- Reduce your risk.

Your next step is to look at sleep. Do you know that you can reduce headache risk by reorganizing your day?

7

The Importance of Sleep

(how reorganizing your day reduces headache risk)

Sleeping better reduces the risk of headaches and improves mood. Hippocrates, the ancient Greek doctor, said that migraine often went away after a deep sleep, and that was five thousand years ago! People with headaches do not sleep for as long as people without headaches. When they do sleep, the quality of sleep is often poor. Worse still, poor sleep makes people with headaches two or three times more likely to feel anxious or depressed.

Sleeping better has a positive effect on mood as well as headache.

If you think your sleep is poor, then you probably have a sleep problem. The most common sleep problem in people with headaches is insomnia. Insomnia means you have difficulty falling asleep, difficulty staying asleep, or a combination of both. Instead of looking for sleeping pills, you should train yourself how to sleep. Retraining yourself to sleep puts you in control and stops your reliance on medication.

The process of retraining is about doing the same thing over and over again around sleep. Developing good sleep habits reduces headache risk by about 30 percent. A lot of this benefit comes from reorganizing your day or your home.

Good sleep habits mean

- relaxing and switching off;
- creating a positive sleep environment; and
- having a set time for getting up—and sticking to it.

Starting to relax means forgetting about the day you just had. Let go of thoughts about tomorrow. If you worry about the next day, it becomes harder to sleep. A good idea is to keep a notepad and pen by your bed. When things come to mind, write them down. Decide to deal with them another day. You cannot do anything about these thoughts while you are asleep. Once you write something down, let the thought go. Your priority is sleep, not sorting out another day's problems.

Biofeedback or relaxation training can reduce alertness and help you sleep without the need for sleeping pills. Using relaxation audio (CDs or MP3 recordings) reduces feelings of tension or anxiety and improves sleep.

You must create a positive sleeping environment. Don't turn the bedroom into a workplace or recreation area. If your bedroom becomes a place where you do everything but sleep, then sleep becomes harder. Don't use your bedroom for work, watching TV, using an iPad, or checking your smartphone. Make a subconscious link between your bedroom and sleeping. Put a note by your bed or on the bedroom door stating, "My bedroom is for sleeping!"

Once you learn to relax, remove distractions from your sleeping area, and set a time for getting up. Choose a waking time that can be kept long term. For example, I usually get up at 6:30 a.m. every day, and I try to be in bed about 11:30 p.m.

The exact number of hours of sleep is not important. Some people feel refreshed with five or six hours, while others need nine or ten hours. We are all different. Your aim is to have a predictable sleep pattern. If you try to get the same amount of sleep each night, you help train your brain to sleep. You need to stick to this waking time seven days a week until you have retrained yourself to sleep. Retraining your brain to sleep can take about three months. You must avoid daytime naps and stick to the same waking time until your sleep pattern improves.

Good sleep habits are difficult at first. When you force yourself to wake at a set time, you increase the desire to sleep later that day. Turn tiredness to your advantage. Stay awake all day until bedtime— this pushes you toward a regular sleep habit. Whatever you do, avoid napping during daytime hours.

When you retrain your sleep, be aware that headaches usually feel worse. Take things easy during these tiring days. If your day involves driving or using machinery, you must avoid these if you are too tired to drive or operate machinery safely.

Invest time and effort in good sleep habits. You get a great return on investment—a better mood and a reduced risk of headaches.

None of this involves taking medication. It is all about organizing yourself: a notepad and pen, clearing your bedroom, and setting an alarm. You just need to stick to it. An example of putting good sleep habits into action is presented in appendix 6.

Next up is how to keep it simple with exercise and diet.

8

Exercise, and What You Eat and Drink

(why you don't need a strict diet)

Common sense and scientific evidence prove that getting active and staying active improve physical and mental health. Maintaining good physical health also reduces your risk of headaches.

Exercise releases your own natural painkillers called endorphins. Endorphins produce happy feelings, and exercise improves mood. Exercise also strengthens your musculoskeletal, cardiovascular, and respiratory systems. If you are not active, then start with walking.

START WITH WALKING

Regular walking reduces the risk of migraine by about 30 percent, an effect similar to any headache prevention medicine. When you walk, you start using inactive muscles. After a short walk, muscles may feel stiff and sore. Over time inactive muscles strengthen, so walking becomes easier and you feel less sore. If you start too fast or go too far, you can get muscle pain, which puts you off trying. You should build up the time and distance you walk.

Walking briskly for thirty minutes three times per week is a good goal. A brisk walk is fast enough to let you just manage to hold a conversation.

You control the amount of walking. Many people with severe headaches are trapped in their own houses. The noise, light, and movement outside are too much to bear. This usually means no activity at all, let alone exercise. The easiest exercise is walking, as no special equipment is required. Anything more intense than walking may feel like you are bringing on headaches or making them worse by overdoing things.

Do not get fooled into thinking that exercise means going to a gym or following an expensive exercise program. Gym and exercise programs can be fun to do, but they are not necessary. It's much better to do something easy that you can control. If you are not walking, then it's by far the best exercise to try.

Step counters can help you to be more active and to motivate you to do more. Try downloading a step counter app for your smartphone or buy a step counter (called a pedometer).

If you never walk outside, start at a target of one hundred steps on day one. Each day add in another one hundred until you get to one thousand steps per day. Then build up by one thousand steps each week until you manage ten thousand steps three days a week. Ideally, for your overall health, aim for ten thousand steps every day.

This produces real benefits to your health and reduces the risk of headaches.

Change your habits to allow you to build more time for walking into your daily routine:

- Park farther from the front door of the store or office.
- Always walk for short journeys under a mile.
- Use public transportation.
- Don't drive to a supermarket, but walk to local shops.

Starting to walk puts you back in control of your own life. Being in control helps you feel less trapped by pain. You are deciding what to do, not your headaches. Whatever you do, start walking to reduce your headache risk and to improve your overall health.

WHAT YOU EAT AND DRINK

No single diet reduces the risk of headache. You may come across diets that claim to cure migraines, but this is not true. Long-term research shows that if you are prone to headaches, then headaches will reappear. Aim to enjoy a healthy, varied diet. Food is one of life's simple pleasures. You should not live in fear of food. If you think what you eat and your headaches are connected, then you must understand the migraine prodrome.

The migraine prodrome is symptoms you get in the days or hours before a headache appears. These symptoms include changes in your appetite and food cravings. In almost every case, the migraine prodrome is making you want the food before the headache appears—it's not the food *causing* the headache. The migraine prodrome is making you want the food, and it can cheat you out of an enjoyable and varied diet.

If a diet claims to cure migraines—beware! A cure is cause-and-effect thinking. You are setting yourself up for disappointment if you start a diet plan in the hope of stopping headaches.

I've not mentioned weight, as it is not clear if losing or gaining weight reduces the risk of migraine or tension-type headaches. It is true that being overweight or very underweight increases the risk of migraines, but it is not clear if changing your weight to a normal range makes headaches better. For overall health and well-being, a normal weight is better. Aim for a weight and lifestyle that make you feel well, but do not go on strict diets with the aim of reducing your risk of headache.

Everyone who has headaches should drink plenty of water each day. A target amount is about three pints (1500 ml) per day. You may need more depending on your local climate. You may need less if you have health problems that require fluid restriction, such as kidney, heart, or pituitary gland disease. Check with your doctor if you are uncertain.

Research shows that people with headache who drink water regularly improve their overall sense of well-being, but it may cause only a small reduction in headache risk. As this is such a simple thing to do, it's silly not to do it, but you cannot expect a major effect on pain.

Many people with headaches invest huge amounts of time research-
ing what they eat and drink. One reason is that diet is something
you can control—you do not need a doctor. A bigger reason is cause-
and-effect thinking. If you think your diet contains triggers or causes
for headaches, then it makes sense to try different diets to see what
happens. But when another headache appears, it can feel like a huge
disappointment.

The Billionaire's Book of Headaches is different. The smart money is
not on finding the perfect diet. It's better to feel safe, accept your
headaches, and take steps to reduce risk. If there is no single diet
that reduces risk, then you are free to enjoy food. Don't frustrate
yourself with endless diets. Stop wasting time on analyzing your diet.
Instead, eat to nourish yourself and to feel well. This puts you back
in control.

The process of analyzing what you eat or do can take over your life.
The next chapter is about why you should break the law of migraine
triggers.

9

The Law of Migraine Triggers

(why it's time you broke the law)

Do any of these sound familiar?

- Don't eat chocolate.
- Don't eat cheese.
- Avoid wearing perfume.
- Don't go out in warm weather.
- Stop drinking coffee.
- Don't eat bread.

These are all instructions to avoid migraine triggers. Migraine triggers are mentioned by every book, blog, or magazine on migraine I've ever seen. It's like the law of migraine.

According to the law of migraine triggers, when you remove all triggers, you should stop headaches. The law of migraine triggers is based on cause-and-effect thinking.

Find the cause—the trigger.

Remove the cause and get the effect—no headaches.

But if you have migraine, then headaches *will* return.

Do not think that avoiding migraine triggers will stop headaches—it's unrealistic. Our Swiss researchers proved that people who get headaches…get headaches. Remember that these people were followed for thirty years and had an average of twenty-two days per year with headaches. Were they trying to avoid triggers? Of course they were! It's been the standard advice since the 1950s.

It is a mistake to invest time and effort in finding that elusive migraine trigger. If you understand the migraine prodrome, then have confidence about breaking the law of migraine triggers.

THE MIGRAINE PRODROME

The migraine prodrome is the set of symptoms, emotions, or sensations in the hours before a migraine headache, including the following:

- Hunger or thirst
- Depression or a sense of doom or irritability
- Elation or feeling full of energy
- Cravings for specific foods
- Fatigue or lethargy
- Intolerance of temperature or humidity

You may know a headache is on its way because you feel migraine prodrome symptoms. Some people cannot put the migraine prodrome into words. It's like a premonition—"I just know a headache is coming."

The migraine prodrome is linked to changes in activity in a part of the brain called the hypothalamus. The hypothalamus controls appetite, thirst, and temperature and influences emotions. Before you get pain, the hypothalamus changes its level of activity, so you get symptoms of the migraine prodrome.

Food cravings are a symptom of the migraine prodrome, so be careful not to think that your headache is caused by specific food. More likely the migraine prodrome is making you want the food. Increased thirst can happen in the migraine prodrome as well, so try not to blame something you drank for causing a migraine. Certain temperatures or humidity levels feel uncomfortable before a headache starts to build. It's not the heat or humidity that causes your headache; your headache is probably making you feel uncomfortable in the heat and humidity due to changes in your hypothalamus from the migraine prodrome.

Our understanding of the migraine prodrome means that migraine triggers are changes in mood, appetite, energy, or perception by changes migraines make to your brain. It's not the trigger causing the migraine but the migraine creating the apparent trigger.

A migraine trigger is easy to believe. It's natural to make a strong connection between what you did just before the onset of a migraine and the migraine headache itself. This is classic cause-and-effect thinking. To make things worse, everybody mentions triggers when you say the word *migraine*. You feel you must record and act on these connections - which is costly and time-consuming. The sad truth is that these connections are likely to be false. Dealing with false connections is a recipe for disappointment.

Migraine triggers make the world a scary place, not somewhere to feel at home. A trigger could appear at any time and give you a headache. The law of migraine triggers is restricting and puts migraines in the center of your life. The law of migraine triggers puts migraines in charge when *you* should be feeling in control. The law of migraine triggers means letting your diet, environment, and daily activity become a threat.

Here are some clues that you are ruled by the law of migraine triggers:

- Do people live by *your* rules to stop *your* migraines?
- Do you read all food labels before eating?
- Have you ever refused to eat something someone prepared for you?
- Have you stopped enjoying yourself with family or friends?
- Do you keep thinking that you will find that elusive trigger?
- Do you stop going outside because of fear of a migraine?

If so, you may be ruled by the law of migraine triggers.

Avoiding migraine triggers is a negative way to live. The process of identifying and removing migraine triggers knows no end. I once read a research paper that described over two hundred different food triggers. After finding and avoiding a migraine trigger, you may feel like you are doing well, like you have solved the migraine problem. Eventually another headache *will* appear—research tells us this. You feel like a failure because your hard work is undone and another headache happened, but you keep on searching.

The search for that elusive trigger steals your attention and effort. If you are not careful, you miss out on life. Don't let fear of headache stop you from doing positive and enjoyable things. Migraine triggers are false connections based on cause-and-effect thinking.

I recommend you abandon this approach, as it frees you to live normally. A good test is to put a date in your diary in the future. If you feel well that day, then try a bit of cheese, bread, or wine and see what happens. Try to "trigger" a headache. As long as you are not feeling like a migraine is already on its way that day, you may be in for a pleasant surprise.

In *The Billionaire's Book of Headaches*, I'm saying to

- feel safe;
- accept your headaches;
- reduce your risk; and
- break the law of migraine triggers.

This is a better strategy. Instead of living in fear, you take control. Live well. Reclaim lost ground. Don't fear your home and environment. Eat a varied diet. Start socializing. Put migraines in the back seat so that you can take control.

Feeling safe, acceptance and risk reduction puts *you* in charge. It's time to break the cruel law of migraine triggers.

10

When It Feels Like Nothing Works

The Billionaire's Book of Headaches shows you how to change your thinking and to reduce your risk of headache. If you put this book into action, you could still have bad headaches and feel like nothing has helped.

You are not alone.

One person in fifty has a headache every day or nearly every day. That's about six million US citizens or 160 million people world-wide with headaches nearly every day. If you struggle with headaches that are not dangerous, then you probably have chronic migraine, the most common and unpleasant reason for daily headaches.

With chronic migraine, there is a constant background pain. On top of this background headache, you get migraines lasting hours or days at a time. The headaches have no real pattern.

With chronic migraine, you experience several non-headache symptoms:

- Migraine prodrome: hunger, thirst, depression, sense of doom, elation, feeling full of energy, cravings for specific foods, fatigue, lethargy, or irritability
- Migraine aura: episodes of flashing lights, tingling (of face, arm, or leg), speech difficulty, dizziness, or vertigo
- Sensory sensitivity: nausea, loss of appetite, pain made worse by looking at light (so you wear dark glasses every day), avoiding noise, avoiding strong smells, feeling uncomfortable when you move or when something touches you

With chronic migraine, pain is unpredictable, although you always feel like looking for a pattern or reason for pain. The symptoms of prodrome, aura, or sensory sensitivity can happen at any time and last for hours, days, or weeks.

With chronic migraine, your head is a ball of chaos.

You will want professional help.

Professional help includes advanced treatments like botulinum toxin injections and nerve stimulators or pain management programs based on cognitive behavioral therapy. If you need professional help, don't just rush out and book the most expensive doctor you can find. Your first step is to feel safe and to make sure you have your thinking straight.

Are you still engaged in cause-and-effect thinking? Are you looking for a cure? Before trying advanced treatments, be realistic. The search for a cure is exhausting, whereas accepting your headaches is a much healthier way to be (see the introduction). Remember to feel safe. When you feel safe, you are free to do whatever you want without fear (see chapter 1). Be certain that you understand your headache and non-headache symptoms—this helps you feel secure (see chapter 2). It sometimes takes several visits to your doctor to know that your symptoms are normal, but when you feel safe, you are free to take whatever steps you wish. Before booking a specialist, remember that the first thing an expensive headache clinic does is to stop all your painkillers, even if that means admitting you to a hospital for several days (see chapter 3).

Are you using medicines correctly? Remember the A + B + C approach of treating a migraine. Do you manage to treat migraines with combinations of medicines before your head is too sore to touch (see chapter 4)? Have you managed to persevere with best doses of at least three different headache prevention medicines for more than three months (see chapter 5)? Do you have a headache diary to show that they did not work?

Remember that physical problems with your neck, jaw, and eyes increase the risk of headache. If you seem to get one-sided headaches or you have very prolonged migraines that last several days, then make sure your neck, jaw, and eyes are OK (see chapter 6).

Are you looking after yourself as well as you can, both physically and mentally? Have you made changes to your sleep habits? A 30 percent reduction in headache is possible just by reorganizing your day (see chapter 7)! Remember that there is no diet proven to cure migraines. It is more important to be active every day and to enjoy a healthy diet. Walking is the best exercise you can undertake if you get headaches. You are in control of how much, how often, and when you walk (see chapter 8).

Finally, break the law of migraine triggers. Don't be a slave to triggers. Live well instead. Test the triggers when you feel well. Your brain is playing tricks on you by linking things you do to getting bad headaches (see chapter 9).

If you have changed your thinking from cause and effect to accept and reduce, or if you feel you have taken reasonable steps to reduce your risk and are still troubled by a lot of headaches, then advanced treatments like botulinum toxin and nerve stimulators may reduce your headache risk.

Advanced treatments are not cures. They reduce your risk of headache. Current technology and scientific knowledge do not offer a cure. If your expectation is too high, then you may be disappointed and feel that your time and money have been wasted. Satisfaction equals experience minus expectation. It is so easy to make what is perfect the enemy of what is good.

If you do not like the risks associated with advanced treatments (all medical procedures carry risks), then your next option is to look at pain management programs.

Pain management programs recognize that your experience of pain is ruled by your moods, emotions, and memories. Pain management programs use psychological techniques, called cognitive behavioral therapy, to change unhelpful thinking into helpful thinking. If you can't change headaches, then change how you think about headaches.

Acceptance of pain is an important part of the pain management process. The true value of pain management programs is to give you a better frame of mind and to let you see simple ways you can regain control. If you know you are safe, then you are free to explore your own ideas.

Professional help is not for everyone, and you may prefer a philosophical approach, which includes religious practice, meditation, and mindfulness practice. Philosophical approaches change your view of the world and help you accept your situation. You end up coping better and feeling more at ease. You must feel free to change in whatever way suits your own personality, perspective, or philosophy, as long as you know you are safe. Philosophical approaches and help with healthier thinking can be found in the useful resources section at the end of this book.

Whatever you do, you still need a doctor you trust when you are dealing with headaches. Family physicians are best placed to balance one illness, symptom, or treatment against another. Family physicians take an overall view of health in a way that specialists cannot. A specialist can help make sure that a headache is not dangerous and propose treatment regimes, but if you cannot access a specialist, then you are not disadvantaged if you know you are safe.

Doctors do not have all the answers, and if you want to try your own approach to headaches, then a good doctor keeps you clear of harm or unnecessary expense. If you like a particular method or idea, then try it for a while and see if your life improves. If it doesn't, don't despair and try another. You should also be on the lookout for clinical trials of new treatments or methods, but beware of cause-and-effect thinking. There are no known cures for headaches, and any treatment, however promising, will only ever reduce the risk of headache.

Conclusions and Next Steps

The Billionaire's Book of Headaches is a different way of thinking and reacting to headaches and contains practical advice to help you avoid common pitfalls.

You need to make sure that you are safe. Then accept that headaches are part of who you are. Understand that many other symptoms go along with migraines, not just pain, such as sensory sensitivity, migraine aura, and migraine prodrome. Feel in control—and feel safe—by knowing about these symptoms.

Work out your best way to treat a migraine with combinations of drugs, and know that drugs to prevent headaches take time to work. Many drug-free options reduce your risk of headache; always pay attention to your neck, jaw, and eyes. You even have a lot to gain by sleeping better.

When you find out more about headache, you will feel in control. When you feel in control, you reduce your risk of headache and rely less on medication. Research proves that people who know more experience fewer headaches and use less medication.

Headaches *will* return at some point, even if you take all reasonable steps to reduce your risk of headache. You need to accept your headache problem and to have a plan of action when a bad headache appears. Remember that your plan of action should include distractions, not just medications.

When all else fails, my suggestion is this:

- Make sure you know your enemy—understand the symptoms of your headache condition.
- Feel safe and get as much reassurance as you can from your doctor.
- Accept that headaches occur, and stop engaging in cause-and-effect thinking.

Then consider professional help, which might be in the form of a pain management program based on cognitive behavioral therapy, or advanced treatments from a specialist headache clinic like botulinum toxin or nerve stimulators. Professional help may include counseling for past trauma or emotional problems that prevent you from coping with pain.

If you don't want professional help, then knowing you are safe provides you with space to discover your own way of coping—whether it's a philosophical approach or a change in lifestyle.

Whatever you do, it is crucial that you change your thinking. If you can't change headaches, then change the way you think about them.

To recap, here are the steps of *The Billionaire's Book of Headaches*:

1. Feel less afraid of pain.
2. Determine your type of headache.
3. Understand why too many painkillers make things worse.

4. Understand how to treat a headache with medicines.
5. Use headache prevention medicines—be smart!
6. Check your neck, jaw, and eyes.
7. Understand the importance of sleep.
8. Understand the importance of exercise and diet.
9. Break the law of migraine triggers.
10. When nothing seems to work, seek professional help.

If you had a billion dollars, this is what you should do.

Remember:

- Feel safe.
- Accept your headaches.
- Reduce risk.

Bibliography

Ahn, A. H. (2010). On the temporal relationship between throbbing migraine pain and arterial pulse. *Headache, 50*(9), 1507–1510.

Ahn, A. H. (2013). Why does increased exercise decrease migraine? *Current Pain Headache Reports, 17*(12), 379.

Akinci, A., Güven, A., Değerliyurt, A., Kibar, E., Mutlu, M., & Citirik, M. (2008). The correlation between headache and refractive errors. *Journal of American Association for Pediatric Ophthalmology and Strabismus, 12*(3), 290–293.

Basu, S., Yoffe, P., Hills, N., & Lustig, R. H. (2013). The relationship of sugar to population-level diabetes prevalence: An econometric analysis of repeated cross-sectional data. *PLoS One, 8*(2), e57873.

Bigal, M. E., Ashina, S., Burstein, R., Reed, M. L., Buse, D., Serrano, D., & Lipton, R. B. (2008). Prevalence and characteristics of allodynia in headache sufferers: A population study. *Neurology, 70*(17), 1525–1533.

Bigal, M. E., & Lipton, R. B. (2009). Excessive opioid use and the development of chronic migraine. *Pain, 142*(3), 179–182.

Blau, J. N., & Thavapalan, M. (1988). Preventing migraine: A study of precipitating factors. *Headache, 28*(7), 481–483.

Breivik, H., Eisenberg, E., & O'Brien, T. (2013). The individual and societal burden of chronic pain in Europe: The case for strategic prioritisation and action to improve knowledge and availability of appropriate care. *BMC Public Health*, *13*, 1229.

British Association for the Study of Headache. (2010). *Guidelines for all healthcare professionals in the diagnosis and management of migraine, tension-type headache, cluster headache, and medication-overuse headache* (3rd ed.). Hull, England: Author.

Burstein R., Collins, B., & Jakubowski, M. (2004). Defeating migraine with triptans: A race against the development of cutaneous allodynia. *Annals of Neurology*, *55*(1), 19–26.

Butler, A. C., Chapman, J. E., Forman, E. M., & Beck, A. T. (2006). The empirical status of cognitive-behavioral therapy: A review of meta-analyses. *Clinical Psychology Review*, *26*(1), 17–31.

Calhoun, A. H., & Ford, S. (2007). Behavioral sleep modification may revert transformed migraine to episodic migraine. *Headache*, *47*(8), 1178–1183.

Ducros, A., Romatet, S., Saint Marc, T., & Allaf, B. (2011). Use of antimigraine treatments by general practitioners. *Headache*, *51*(7), 1122–1131.

Fordyce, W. E. (1984). Behavioural science and chronic pain. *Postgraduate Medical Journal*, *60*(710), 865–868.

Freitag, F. G., Lake III, A., Lipton, R., Cady, R., Diamond, S., & Silberstein, S. (2004). Inpatient treatment of headache: An evidence-based assessment. *Headache, 44*(4), 342–360.

Giffin, N. J., Ruggiero, L., Lipton, R. B., Silberstein, S. D., Tvedskov, J. F., Olesen, J.,...Macrae, A. (2003). Premonitory symptoms in migraine: An electronic diary study. *Neurology, 60*(6), 935–940.

Gil-Gouveia, R. (2014). Headache from the doctors' perspective. *European Neurology, 71*(3–4), 157–164.

Gil-Gouveia, R., & Martins, I. P. (2002). Headaches associated with refractive errors: Myth or reality? *Headache, 42*(4), 256–262.

Gonzalez, Y. M., Schiffman, E., Gordon, S. M., Seago, B., Truelove, E. L., Slade, G., & Ohrbach, R. (2011). Development of a brief and effective temporomandibular disorder pain screening questionnaire: Reliability and validity. *Journal of the American Dental Association, 142*(10), 1183–1191.

Gunes, A., Demirci, S., Tok, L., Tok, O., Koyuncuoglu, H., & Yurekli, V. A. (2015). Refractive errors in patients with migraine headache. *Seminars in Ophthalmology, 31*(5), 1–3.

Harle, D. E., & Evans, B. J. (2006). The correlation between migraine headache and refractive errors. *Optometry & Vision Science, 83*(2), 82–87.

Hauge, A. W., Kirchmann, M., & Olesen, J. (2010). Trigger factors in migraine with aura. *Cephalalgia, 30*(3), 346–353.

Hayes, S. C. (2004). Acceptance and commitment therapy, relational frame theory, and the third wave of behavioral and cognitive therapies. *Behavior Therapy, 35*(4), 639–665.

Horton, B. T., & Peters, G. A. (1963). Clinical manifestations of excessive use of ergotamine preparations and management of withdrawal effect: Report of 52 cases. *Headache, 2*(4), 214–227.

Katsarava, Z., Fritsche, G., Muessig, M., Diener, H. C., & Limmroth, V. (2001). Clinical features of withdrawal headache following overuse of triptans and other headache drugs. *Neurology, 57*(9), 1694–1698.

Kindelan-Calvo, P., Gil-Martínez, A., Paris-Alemany, A., Pardo-Montero, J., Muñoz-García, D., Angulo-Díaz-Parreño, S., & La Touche, R. (2014). Effectiveness of therapeutic patient education for adults with migraine: A systematic review and meta-analysis of randomized controlled trials. *Pain Medicine, 15*(9), 1619–1636.

Kristoffersen, E. S., & Lundqvist, C. (2014). Medication-overuse headache: A review. *Journal of Pain Research, 7*, 367–378.

Linde, K., Allais, G., Brinkhaus, B., Manheimer, E., Vickers, A., & White, A. R. (2009). Acupuncture for migraine prophylaxis. *Cochrane Database of Systematic Reviews, 1*, CD001218.

Mansi, S., Milosavljevic, S., Baxter, G. D., Tumilty, S., & Hendrick, P. (2014). A systematic review of studies using pedometers as an intervention for musculoskeletal diseases. *BMC Musculoskeletal Disorders, 15,* 231.

Mantyh, P. W. (2014). The neurobiology of skeletal pain. *European Journal of Neuroscience, 39*(3), 508–519.

Martin, P. R. (2010). Managing headache triggers: Think "coping" not "avoidance." *Cephalalgia, 30*(5), 634–637.

Martin, P. R., & MacLeod, C. (2009). Behavioral management of headache triggers: Avoidance of triggers is an inadequate strategy. *Clinical Psychology Review, 29*(6), 483–495.

Mathew, N. T., Kurman, R., & Perez, F. (1990). Drug induced refractory headache—Clinical features and management. *Headache, 30*(10), 634–638.

May, A. (2017). Understanding migraine as a cycling brain syndrome: reviewing the evidence from functional brain imaging. *Neurological Sciences, 38*(1), 125-130.

Moseley, G. L., & Butler, D. S. (2015). 15 years of explaining pain—The past, present, and future. *Journal of Pain, 16*(9), 807–813.

Mo'tamedi, H., Rezaiemaram, P., & Tavallaie, A. (2012). The effectiveness of a group-based acceptance and commitment additive therapy on rehabilitation of female outpatients with chronic headache: Preliminary findings reducing 3 dimensions of headache impact. *Headache*, *52*(7), 1106–1119.

Mulleners, W. M., McCrory, D. C., & Linde, M. (2015). Antiepileptics in migraine prophylaxis: An updated Cochrane review. *Cephalalgia*, *35*(1), 51–62.

Nijs, J., Paul van Wilgen, C., Van Oosterwijck, J., van Ittersum, M., & Meeus, M. (2011). How to explain central sensitization to patients with "unexplained" chronic musculoskeletal pain: Practice guidelines. *Manual Therapy*, *16*(5), 413–418.

Ornello, R., Ripa, P., Pistoia, F., Degan, D., Tiseo, C., Carolei, A., & Sacco, S. (2015). Migraine and body mass index categories: A systematic review and meta-analysis of observational studies. *Journal of Headache and Pain*, *16*(1), 27.

Pageler, L., Katsarava, Z., Diener, H. C., & Limmroth, V. (2008). Prednisone vs. placebo in withdrawal therapy following medication overuse headache. *Cephalalgia*, *28*(2), 152–156.

Pini, L. A., Cicero, A. F., & Sandrini, M. (2001). Long-term follow-up of patients treated for chronic headache with analgesic overuse. *Cephalalgia*, *21*(9), 878–883.

Rabe, K., Pageler, L., Gaul, C., Lampl, C., Kraya, T., Foerderreuther, S.,…Katsarava, Z. (2013). Prednisone for the treatment of withdrawal headache in patients with medication overuse headache: A randomized, double-blind, placebo-controlled study. *Cephalalgia, 33*(3), 202–207.

Scher, A.I., Rizzoli, P.B., Loder, E.W. (2017). Medication overuse headache. An entrenched idea in need of scrutiny. *Neurology, 89 (12), 1296-1304.*

Schoenen, J., Vandersmissen, B., Jeangette, S., Herroelen, L., Vandenheede, M., Gérard, P.,…Magis, D. (2013). Migraine prevention with a supraorbital transcutaneous stimulator: A randomized controlled trial. *Neurology, 80*(8), 697–704.

Schulte, L. H., Jurgens, T. P., & May, A. (2015). Photo-, osmo- and phonophobia in the premonitory phase of migraine: Mistaking symptoms for triggers? *Journal of Headache and Pain, 16*(1), 14.

Smith, T. R. (2002). Low-dose tizanidine with nonsteroidal anti-inflammatory drugs for detoxification from analgesic rebound headache. *Headache, 42*(3), 175–177.

Speciali, J. G., & Dach, F. (2015). Temporomandibular dysfunction and headache disorder. *Headache, 55*(Suppl 1), 72–83.

Spigt, M., Weerkamp, N., Troost, J., van Schayck, C. P., & Knottnerus, J. A. (2012). A randomized trial on the effects of regular water intake in patients with recurrent headaches. *Family Practice, 29*(4), 370–375.

Sprouse-Blum, A. S., Gabriel, A. K., Brown, J. P., & Yee, M. H. (2013). Randomized controlled trial: Targeted neck cooling in the treatment of the migraine patient. *Hawaii Journal of Medicine and Public Health*, 72(7), 237–241.

Teigen, L., & Boes, C. J. (2015). An evidence-based review of oral magnesium supplementation in the preventive treatment of migraine. *Cephalalgia*, 35(10), 912—922.

Vanderpol, J., Bishop, B., Matharu, M., & Glencorse, M. (2015). Therapeutic effect of intranasal evaporative cooling in patients with migraine: A pilot study. *Journal of Headache and Pain*, 16, 5.

Wallston, B. D., & Wallston, K. A. (1978). Locus of control and health: A review of the literature. *Health Education Monographs*, 6(2), 107–117.

Woolf, C. J. (2011). Central sensitization: Implications for the diagnosis and treatment of pain. *Pain*, 152(Suppl 3), S2–S15.

Zanchin, G., Maggioni, F., Granella, F., Rossi, P., Falco, L., & Manzoni, G. C. (2001). Self-administered pain-relieving manoeuvres in primary headaches. *Cephalalgia*, 21(7), 718–726.

Zeeberg, P., Olesen, J., & Jensen, R. (2006). Discontinuation of medication overuse in headache patients: Recovery of therapeutic responsiveness. *Cephalalgia*, 26(10), 1192–1198.

Zidverc-Trajkovic, J., Pekmezovic, T., Jovanovic, Z., Pavlovic, A., Mijajlovic, M., Radojicic, A., & Sternic, N. (2007). Medication overuse headache: Clinical features predicting treatment outcome at 1-year follow-up. *Cephalalgia, 27*(11), 1219–1225.

Websites

The companion website for *The Billionaire's Book of Headaches* is Severe Headache Expert: www.severe-headache-expert.com

Professional and Patient Support Organizations

The Migraine Association of Ireland: www.migraine.ie

The Migraine Trust (United Kingdom): www.migrainetrust.org

Migraine Action (United Kingdom): www.migraine.org.uk

International Headache Society: www.ihs-headache.org

The American Headache Society: www.americanheadachesociety.org

British Association for Study of Headache: www.bash.org.uk

Lifting The Burden: The Global Campaign against Headache: www.l-t-b.org

Self-Help Blogs

Teri Robert's Health Guide
http://www.healthcentral.com/profiles/c/123

Lisa Jacobson's The Daily Migraine
www.thedailymigraine.com/

Philosophical Approaches
The Lightning Process by Phil Parker
https://lightningprocess.com/

Mindfulness Help for Pain, Depression, and Anxiety
Headspace App
https://www.headspace.com/

Good Sleep Habits Course
Sleepio
https://www.sleepio.com/

Clinical Trials Registers
US-Based Global Register
https://clinicaltrials.gov/

European Union Trials
https://www.clinicaltrialsregister.eu/

Appendixes

Appendix 1
Action Points

The following list of action points will help you reduce your risk of headaches.

Remember that you must seek medical advice if you have a new onset of headaches or a new type of headache that is unusually severe.

Once I know I am safe:

1. I can accept that I will get headaches. YES / NO
2. I need to reduce risk, not cure, headaches. YES / NO
3. I can see that migraine pain is a false alarm. YES / NO
4. I understand which headache types I have. YES / NO
5. I have dealt with overuse of painkillers. YES / NO
6. I know to treat a migraine attack (A + B + C). YES / NO
7. I'll be smart with headache prevention medicine. YES / NO
8. I've seen a physiotherapist or osteopath. YES / NO
9. I have asked my dentist about my jaw. YES / NO
10. I have visited an optician. YES / NO
11. I walk ten thousand steps per day. YES / NO
12. I drink three pints (1500 ml) of water each day. YES / NO
13. Good sleep habits are now a priority. YES / NO
14. I want to enjoy food and eat well. YES / NO
15. I understand the law of migraine triggers. YES / NO

Appendix 2
How to Stop Painkillers: A Diary of Someone Overusing Acetaminophen

Hi. My name is Yvonne, and I've been getting migraines since I was fifteen years old. I'm now thirty-three and have been getting a headache nearly every day for the last six months. About once a week, I'm in bed for a whole day with a headache.

When my doctor explained to me that taking painkillers every day was maybe making things worse, I was surprised. I was buying acetaminophen every week and taking about six to eight tablets every day. My doctor told me to stop all acetaminophen and gave me a prescription for an anti-inflammatory medicine to take for two weeks (it was called naproxen).

I was frightened about stopping painkillers, as it felt like I was asking for trouble—the headaches would surely get worse! I stopped the acetaminophen on the same day I started the naproxen. My head didn't feel too bad. The next day was worse. When I woke up, it felt like my head was throbbing, and another bad headache seemed like it was on its way.

I was so tempted to take the acetaminophen but knew I should not. I tried to distract myself and to not think too much about the painkillers. I went for a walk for a half hour, which was good. My head continued to throb—I'd say about a 6 or 7 out of 10 for the next four days. I continued to take the naproxen, and my head would still throb and feel like another headache was not far away, but I was determined not to go back to the painkillers.

By the beginning of the second week, my head felt a bit dull, but not so much throbbing, and the feeling to take painkillers wasn't so strong. My worst day was at the end of week two, when I spent a day in bed with a severe headache, like a really bad migraine. I knew all I could do was sleep and rest until the pain passed. I did not want to give in and take the acetaminophen again.

It's now eight weeks since I stopped acetaminophen, and I have had only two bad headaches in all that time. My head feels a lot clearer now.

If you are going to stop painkillers, my advice is to be determined and to stick with the plan. You also need to know that headaches will take time to settle and that stopping acetaminophen or any other painkiller is not a cure. Some headaches still seem to happen, but I think I am a lot healthier not having to take painkillers all the time.

I've always hated taking medicine, and it's such a relief to feel like I've managed to cut it back.

Appendix 3
Treating a Headache Using A + B + C

Here's how someone treated a headache using the A + B + C approach.

The person went to the doctor and received a supply of naproxen 500 mg (group A), sumatriptan 100 mg (group B), and metoclopramide 10 mg (group C).

10.30 a.m. Migraine starts; head not sore to touch and no nausea

Took naproxen 500 mg *and* sumatriptan 100 mg (A + B)
Slept for an hour (distraction)

3.15 p.m. Still quite sore, feeling nauseated

Took naproxen 500 mg *and* sumatriptan 100 mg *and* metoclopramide 10 mg (A + B + C)
Told myself that I'm going to be OK
Went for a short walk to distract myself

11:00 p.m. Still feeling pain at about 4 out of 10 severity, less nausea

Went to bed
Listened to relaxing music (another distraction)
Tried to sleep[5]

---

5 Some people with occasional, very severe migraine can use a mild sleeping pill one or two times each month to bring on sleep if painkillers have not worked. Sleep has long been known to help relieve migraines.

7:00 a.m. The next day, the pain is at 2 out of 10

    Got up and went for short walk (distraction)
    Took naproxen 500 mg (group A painkiller)

Bedtime, next day: Head feels OK; has been a tiring day

Appendix 4
Printable Three-Month Headache Diary

Month	1	2	3	4	5	6	7	8	9	10	11	12	13	14	15	16
Pain score																
Painkillers																
	17	18	19	20	21	22	23	24	25	26	27	28	29	30	31	
Pain score																
Painkillers																
Month	1	2	3	4	5	6	7	8	9	10	11	12	13	14	15	16
Pain score																
Painkillers																
	17	18	19	20	21	22	23	24	25	26	27	28	29	30	31	
Pain score																
Painkillers																
Month	1	2	3	4	5	6	7	8	9	10	11	12	13	14	15	16
Pain score																
Painkillers																
	17	18	19	20	21	22	23	24	25	26	27	28	29	30	31	
Pain score																
Painkillers																

Enter a number from 0 to 10 for each day with headache (0 is no pain, and 10 is the worst imaginable pain). Also note if you took painkillers by placing an *X* in the appropriate column. Make any other comments on the back of this sheet.

Appendix 5
Finding the Best Dose of a Headache Prevention Medicine

Here's an example of finding a best dose of a drug called topiramate. The maximum dose used in most people is 50 mg twice a day, but up to 200 mg twice daily can be used.

The person using the drug has a supply of 25 mg tablets from his pharmacist.

The instruction from the pharmacist is to start at 25 mg once a day and to increase every week until a maximum of 50 mg twice daily is reached.

Somewhere between 25 mg once daily and 50 mg twice daily is this person's best dose.

Here's what this person did:

May 1 to May 7
Took 25 mg every morning, felt OK. No major headaches but felt some pins and needles in my fingers. My doctor told me to expect this, as it means the topiramate is in my system.

May 8 to May 15
Increased to 25 mg every morning and 25 mg at night. Still getting some pins and needles. Had a headache on May 11, which went away by the next day. Sometimes think I'm a bit slow to think of the right word.

May 16 to May 23

Increased to 50 mg in the morning and 25 mg at night. The pins and needles are more obvious. Feel tired and can't think of the right words again. Phoned my doctor, who said these sound like side effects. Not sure I could take any more topiramate but will try the next step.

May 24 and May 25

Increased to 50 mg morning and night. Couldn't get the right words and felt really intense pins and needles. Don't think I could manage this dose for another twelve weeks!

May 26

Phoned my doctor, who said to reduce back to 50 mg in the morning and 25 mg at night. This is my best dose, as it's the most I can tolerate.

May 27 to May 30

Stayed on 50 mg in the morning and 25 mg at night. Still some pins and needles, but I can manage this. Word-finding problem not so noticeable.

May 31 for next twelve weeks

Managed to stay on 50 mg in the morning and 25 mg at night. My diary shows that the number of headaches reduced from about eight per month to five per month.

In this case the best dose was 50 mg of topiramate in the morning and 25 mg at night.

The usual recommended dose is 50 mg twice a day. So in this case the best dose for this person is less, but it still had the desired effect of reducing the risk of headaches.

Appendix 6
Good Sleep Habits in Practice: An Example

Clear your bedroom of distractions.

Decide on your getting-up time.

Set an alarm for your getting-up time.

Avoid caffeine (e.g., tea, coffee, fizzy drinks) after midday.

Late in the evening, when you want to sleep, go to bed and try to fall asleep.

If, after turning over or repositioning yourself two or three times, you are still unable to asleep, get up and leave the bedroom.

Return to bed only when you feel tired enough to try to sleep again. (You may need to keep on getting up and trying again and again for several hours.)

You will eventually fall asleep, even if it's nearly 6:00 a.m.

Get up when your alarm goes off, no matter how tired you feel. (Do not be tempted to hit the snooze button or to sleep in. You are trying to train your body and mind into a regular sleeping habit.)

Do everything you can to stay awake all day. Avoid napping during the day at all costs.

When you get close to your set bedtime, go back to the beginning and start again.

Doses should always be checked in a prescribing formulary or with your own doctor or pharmacist.

Dr. Raeburn Forbes and Forbes Neurology Services Ltd. will not be liable for any consequence alleged as a result of reading or acting upon this material in print or online. Written health information is not a substitute for proper medical care. A qualified medical professional should always be consulted about symptoms causing concern. In the context of headaches, a new onset of headache requires medical attention, and the contents of this book do not apply if you have never sought medical advice for a headache symptom.

Published in 2017 by Forbes Neurology Services Ltd., Newtownabbey, United Kingdom. UK Registered Limited Company NI608770.

Index